Short 'N Sweet:

The 20-Minute Home Workout Solution For Busy Parents

DANIEL MUNDAY

For Emily and Jade

Thank You

Thank you to the DPMers who have allowed me to run a successful business since 2005 and to my wife Bronwyn for believing and supporting me.

Also a massive thanks to you, for investing in this book, and for reading it. Make sure you actually do something with the information you've got in your hands!

And remember, if you have any questions about any of these workouts, or if you'd like to look into any potential training options that we might be able to do for you, you can always send me an email - daniel@dpmtransformation.com

Contents

Introduction

This book isn't supposed to sit on your shelf and gather dust. It's a workbook. So write in it. Make notes.

Use the program templates and other free stuff on the dedicated Short 'N Sweet page of my website to maximise your success.

dpmworkout.com

This is also a short book on purpose. Why? So the message doesn't get lost.

Guess what? I know exactly how you feel right now.

How? Because busy Sydney women (and some fellas) just like you, have been coming to DPM since 2005 to discover how to finally lose the 5-10kgs that seem to have crept on, despite trying hard to 'be good' and exercising for hours on end without getting anywhere.

So, if you're over feeling tired, grumpy or bloated and sick of bouncing from one diet to another, you're in the right spot.

But before you start, I strongly advise you to get clearance from your doctor. Especially if you're not currently doing any exercise, or if you have an injury.

I also strongly recommend getting a qualified trainer for a session to show you how to do the exercises properly.

Or, invest in the full follow-along-at-home workout videos where I do it with you in real-time. Otherwise, at the very least, look at the demonstration videos for the correct technique.

Here's a little legal nitty-gritty: By following these workouts, or any information in this book, you agree to waive Daniel Munday and DPM Performance of any responsibility caused by injury that may result.

Now, before you get into the workouts, I want to share a couple of articles to help you on your journey. Read them, absorb what resonates and use it to fuel you towards what you want to achieve.

You'll also discover the stories of busy mums, and even a time-poor dad, all wanting to do something to get on the right track.

The one thing they all have in common is they took action. You can achieve impressive results without having to take too much time-out from your job and family.

Don't believe me? Check out the Short 'N Sweet success stories in this book, plus before and after photos and video testimonials that you'll find all over my website dpmtransformation.com

Want Me To Do All The Workouts With You?

Well, granted, I won't physically be in your home doing these workouts with you over the next six months, but I can offer you the next best thing.

What if I could demonstrate every month's workout in real-time? So that you know exactly how to do the exercises as you're going through them. It's just like having a personal trainer in your home as you do the workout.

What if you could watch the different exercise variations for beginners or the advanced versions? And all you had to do was click on a link for that particular workout? Would that be something you'd be interested in?

It'll give you peace of mind, and motivation that only comes with me doing these workouts with you and providing the right timing for each exercise. All in the comfort of your own home. You'd be crazy to give this a miss.

These videos, and more, come with the DPM All-In Package that you'll see in more details on the next page.

Sure, if you decide against this option you'll still have access to each of the short video demonstrations available on the Short 'N Sweet resources page, but you won't have me walking you through each workout, and providing the appropriate coaching and timing cues.

Six Super Secrets To Skinny Jeans Success

Warning: These secrets will take you from dragging your heels and hiding under baggy clothes to energised and gorgeous just by following these six simple steps.

1. Break The Rules For Faster Results

Never listen to what the mainstream media and big brand companies tell you is the 'right way to eat.' You know the old food pyramid that you see on most packaged foods? It recommends you base your diet around breads, cereals and dairy. Sound familiar?

To be honest, wheat and dairy (even if you aren't coeliac) don't go down well with most people. It can leave them feeling sluggish, bloated and with poor skin. That doesn't mean you can't have them, just limit them, especially if you notice your body doesn't respond well to them.

They also tell you to eat low-fat, or no fat foods because fat is bad. We've been told this for years. This is wrong. Because, fat actually fills you up, so you end up eating less food than you otherwise would when you eat low-fat foods.

Plus, when fat is taken out of foods something has to be added (yucky artificial sweeteners that only make you eat more) because, as well as filling people up, fat gives food taste.

Don't believe me? Try it for yourself for a week and see if you notice the difference. And then when you do, imagine how much that can change over the course of a month or longer?

2. Eat Your Favourite Foods

Yep definitely! In fact 'cheating' is actually going to help you achieve your new toned and shapely body. For the best results, limit yourself to three to four 'cheat meals' each week where you can eat absolutely anything that you want.

Yes, including bread, pasta, cake, slices and even wine. Whatever your thing is! This is because it resets your body's metabolism to go back to fat-burning mode. This is a very simplified view of the process but it works. Some people even report looking leaner the day after a cheat meal.

3. Bye, Bye Boring Cardio and Hours In The Gym

You can achieve better results in less time without spending hours and hours each week slaving away on the treadmill. The truth is that even a short workout that's as little as 20-minutes in length or less (like you'll find in this book) can be more effective than slogging away on the treadmill for an hour day in, day out.

As soon as you stop running on the treadmill, or any boring long distance cardio, your fat burning stops. After doing a high-intensity circuit, your metabolism is kick-started and you're burning way more calories (body fat!) for the next 24-hours.

Some studies even indicate up to a 48-hour window of excess fat burn. The key is to select exercises that maximise your fat burn. That means you need to hit as many muscle groups at the same time (like squats, push-ups, rows and lunges). Just the same sort of stuff we use here.

4. Add This Food To Your Daily Food Plan

Coconut Oil is a bit of a wonder product. It can help increase your metabolism so you burn fat faster. Who doesn't want that? It builds immunity and is great for your skin. There's not much it can't do. Add it to your black coffee, herbal teas and use with cooking instead of other oils.

I also recommend eating it straight from the jar during your initial weight loss phase as weird as that may sound. It's usually a solid white substance in cooler weather (have up to a quarter of a teaspoon) or when it's hotter, and it melts, have a full teaspoon.

5. Avoid The Number One Shortcut Everyone Tries To Make

One of the biggest mistakes most people make is that they try to burn the candle at both ends, yet still expect to see results. It makes it pretty much impossible to lose those stubborn kilos if you don't get enough sleep.

Try to aim for at least seven hours of sleep each night if possible. Obviously, it's not always possible with kids, but do your best. Any less and you're limiting your body's ability to recover, burn fat and mentally unwind. However, if you can't get that, do your best. The more the better.

To help switch your brain off, try and avoid phones/computers/work before bed to wind your brain down. Use relaxation techniques if you struggle with this - breathing, reading, bath/shower or whatever works. I find reading in bed helps switch my mind off from everything else going on.

6. Invest In Someone To Keep You Accountable

Either train with a friend or invest in a trainer who aligns with your goals and personality. I know a good one if you're looking...

The important thing to remember is not everyone will be a good fit for you and your needs/injury requirements. So be sure to find someone who gets you and is the right fit.

Always choose experience and someone who guarantees their results even if they're slightly more expensive. Remember, you get what you pay for!

And if you do decide to go it alone, this book is the perfect start for you, with a complete six-month program laid out for you. Especially when you invest in the follow-along-at-home video demonstrations and Re-Set program that come with the All-In package.

The Definitive Guide To Why Gyms Are Terrifying

Not too long ago, I was sent an article by a client titled "The definitive guide to why gyms are terrifying if you are not 22 years old".

It sums up why I don't like training in gyms. There are too many show ponies and that doof-doof music, or whatever the cool kids call it these days, kills me.

By the way, you know you're getting old when the music the 'young kids' listen to is nothing like it used to be, and you pull out the old 'back in my day when they used to make real music' line.

Plus, all these fancy machines are nowhere near as effective as using your own bodyweight or a couple of resistance tubes or kettlebells.

Give me the great outdoors any day. Even in winter, training outside is great once you get past the early morning chill. What better way to get back on track then to exercise outside in a park getting some vitamin D and overlooking some pretty nice water views?

So if you need a bit of reassurance that you're not the only one who feels intimated walking into a gym filled with people who look young enough to be your child, then you can be comforted in the fact that you're not alone.

And if you're wondering, a DPM session is nothing like that. You'll be among 'your people'. Ones that get you. And don't expect you to do your makeup and take that duck-faced selfie shot halfway through a workout. Because if you don't post your workout on Instagram it didn't happen right?

Not here. All you have to do is take the first step. And for you, that first step is following these workouts and doing them outside or in your lounge room. The main thing is find what works for you.

What's The Best Time Of The Day To Workout?

Truth be told, there isn't a 'best' time of day. It depends on you! The best time of the day to workout is when you're going to do it. Simple really isn't it? Some people perform better in the mornings. Some people would rather walk over broken glass than be disturbed before the sun rises.

Some are suited to lunch hours to give them a break, or an excuse to get out from behind the desk. Some need to get it done after the kids go to bed at night.

So, as you can see it's all pretty subjective. I could spin you some BS about it being scientifically more effective if you exercised when the sun was at a certain co-ordinate in the sky because it means you get that extra 1% out of your workout.

But really, do it when you can. Just get it done. The one thing I do tend to find however, is that a large majority of busy people prefer to get it done early. Before their day starts. I like that because it means nothing else can get in the way.

You can't get stuck at your desk because your boss wants a thousand things done before you leave. You can't get a call that your kid is sick and have to pick them up.

Plus you get the benefit of the 'kick-start' to the day. The feel good feeling that you get after you've exercised. The good hormones are released in your brain.

You're less stressed. You're possibly not even as tired. You're not craving that coffee hit so you don't kill someone who looks at you the wrong way. Although that first coffee still does taste good!

By the way at DPM, you won't be the most unfit one there with everyone making jokes behind your back. We're not some gym junkie cross-fit class where you have to be under-30 and in peak condition with a hipster beard. We're all in it together in a friendly atmosphere.

How Often?

I've been asked a few questions over the years, as I'm sure you can imagine. But a big question that I'm always asked is how often do you train?

See, some people might have the impression that I train every day and love it. And that you should too. Nope.

Some others have the idea that all I do is stand around and tell others what to do. Not that either. Just sometimes...

See, the truth is I used to train every day – well six days a week. And twice a day at that. Guess I was a bit obsessed, but that was back in the day when I was in my 20s with all the time in the world on my hands.

I was single, no kids and obviously not much of a life either to be able to do that. I kind of went from one extreme to the other, I was out on the drink all the time or training just a few years earlier.

Nowadays, like you, I've got a tonne of other things I'd rather be doing than exercising. Like spending time with Emily and Jade for one.

Plus, paying for all the old injuries I used to ignore and not rehab properly makes it a hell of a lot harder to move around now.

To be honest, I'd rather be spending time with the family. Or sitting on the lounge watching footy or basketball, although I do like my workout time.

So how often do you train each week? Are you worried that it isn't enough? To be honest, anything is better than nothing.

Now it's time to answer the question for me. Mostly I do a bodyweight workout two or three days a week. Sometimes I use tubes, rollers and bands. You'll find out more about them in the resources part of this book.

But I also like to walk. And lately I've been doing it more often. It gets me out of the house and lets me clear my head and listen to a podcast. In fact, plenty of ideas I've implemented for this book came from these walks.

The workouts that I do are 20 minutes tops most days. Does that surprise you? Or make you feel more comfortable about your training?

I hope so. I've come to realise that you don't have to train every day to get results.

You don't have to commit hours each week. Especially when you follow what works - just like the DPM sessions you'll find in this book.

I take the same approach. I know exercise isn't the favourite thing you'd rather be doing each week when you have a hundred things on your to-do list.

Sure, I get incidental exercise in addition to my regular walks, and I encourage you to do so too. I'm sure you already do lugging the kids around everywhere and in your day-to-day jobs.

But the days of training for hours and hours just to get any results are long gone. The beauty of less time to train just means when you do it, you do it properly. Just like anything.

Human nature means we get more done if we have a short deadline in which to do something. And the same goes for exercise. It means we've got to train efficiently and only do exercises that are going to give us the biggest bang for our buck.

I encourage you to do the same. Does that make sense?

Is It Really Enough?

In the previous chapter, I talked about how sometimes less is more. Especially when it comes to the number of days you work out. Now I'm going to address something that I get asked a lot. Especially when someone is looking to find out more about what we do here at Team DPM.

Is 30 minutes for our face-to-face sessions (or less for the home workouts) enough time to workout? Will it help you get back into your skinny jeans and lose that stubborn flabby tummy that you can't seem to shift?

Is that time frame, especially when you take out a few minutes for warm-up and stretching down at the end, effective? And I get that. But, the short answer is definitely*. However, there's a big asterisk there for a reason. You have to select the right exercises and train at the right intensity.

Here's a case in point. How many times have you seen that gym bunny or skinny guy, who walks around like he's carrying a couple of invisible beer kegs under his arms, just spend the majority of their one-hour workout staring in the mirror? Pretty much every single person, every single day. Am I right?

And, how many times have you seen that same person just focus on exercises that use only one muscle group at a time – like abs and doing a thousand crunches. Or, the typical gym poser bloke who spends an hour doing arm curls and bench presses. To get those mirror muscles on point. Curls for the girls right?

I'll let you in on a little secret. I hate crunches and I'd say we haven't done them for about 10 years in a DPM session.

Our 30-minute sessions, and the workouts in this book that are even shorter are plenty of time, if you're using exercises that combine multiple muscles at once. And, when you use a structured timer-based format that minimises your downtime you get more done in less time. So yes, shorter sessions are definitely effective.

Provided it's done the right way. The DPM way. Sure, you can go for longer if you have the time (and like some of our group sessions are), but it's not essential.

What's The Best Type Of Workout?

The best workout is whatever one you'll do. It's true. But it's got to include a couple of things:

1) Something that's going to get your heart rate up.

Now, this is obviously going to be dependent on where you are now. If you're starting out, getting your heart rate up might be something as simple as a walk. Or, if you've been doing this training caper for a while now, it'll need to be something a bit more in-depth.

2) That means you need to pick exercises that work a number of body parts at the same time. So stuff like push-ups, deadlifts, squats, and rows are all perfect examples.

Other bodyweight examples that you'll find us doing at DPM include stuff like Blast Offs, Tabletop Holds and so forth. Even midsection exercises like Up and Overs and Side to Side Hovers hit pretty much every muscle in that midsection of yours.

And when we do any of the hover variations you'll notice that we sometimes use a roller, to once again maximise everywhere it hits.

Boxing is also a great full body workout when you do it properly. Otherwise, it's just your arms getting smashed if you're not using your hips to power your punch.

That's the secret. Short 'N Sweet right? The real trick is creating a structured workout to achieve your results in the short sessions you do a few times a week.

And, that's where I come in at DPM. Whether that's for face-to-face sessions or via follow-along-at-home workouts like the ones you'll find in this book.

The goal is to take all that confusion out of everything. And that's when the results start to accumulate - providing you do the work!

You Could

You could start today. Or you could put things off because 'it's too hot' or 'too cold'. You could start tomorrow. Or you could put it off saying I'll start Monday – got a busy week on.

You could kid yourself that your pants aren't feeling tighter then they may have been only a few short months ago. Or you could take the 'something's got to change because I'm not getting any fatter' approach.

Because the cold hard truth is that the mirror isn't going to lie to you. It's like Snow White where the magic mirror on the wall always tells the truth. It's the cold hard dose of reality.

However with avoidance of reality, comes the truth that things only get worse.

You could 'wing it' and go it alone. Or you could follow the foolproof plan that has worked for a ridiculous number of busy women (and even the blokes too), some of which you'll find in this book.

Want proof? Check out the stories you'll read within these pages and on the DPM website dpmtransformation.com

They're all busy people just like you. But they made the commitment and did the work. It doesn't take long. No, you don't have to promise me your first born (I'm happy with my kids thanks!) or commit hours and hours. It's easy to follow and in minimal time.

You could just skip this book and do nothing. Or you could do the hard thing and start. Take the chance. Back yourself.

With the right game plan even if the circumstances aren't perfect (and let's be honest, the circumstances will never be perfect) it can work for you. What have you got to lose?

Things will get easier. I promise you. The hardest part is always starting, and once the first few workouts are crossed-off, then it just becomes the new normal. Trust me.

Ever Feel Like Giving Up?

Ever get that feeling when it all seems a bit too much? You know, just one of those days when you're wondering what on earth did you get yourself into.

Maybe it's your job. Maybe it's that realisation when you stare in the mirror and it suddenly hits you that you're not 21 anymore and you've got more flabby bits that you never imagined possible. Maybe it's that pair of jeans that just don't fit anymore.

I know how you feel. It's scary. It reminds me of the first time I went to work overseas. A mate got me a job as a camp counsellor in the States. He'd done it for the past two summers and as soon as I'd finished uni I told him to hook me up. I was 21. It was my first solo trip overseas.

My mate wasn't getting there until a few days after I did. I'll never forget my first day at the camp. I was scared and wondering 'What the hell have I got myself into?'

I was a long way from home. I didn't know anyone. I was in a strange country, stuck literally in the middle of nowhere. All in the days before smart phones and internet at your fingertips. I had to line up for the good old dial up access at the one computer the camp had!

Well, it sure felt like in the middle of nowhere. The camp was at the top of a mountain with the nearest town in Alabama a 20-minute drive away. The only thing to do was go to Wal-Mart or the movies because it was a dry county and the nearest bar was 45 minutes away.

I was having regrets. You know how it feels. I was lonely and apprehensive. But you know what? I stuck it out.

Sure, it helped that my mate got there a few days later but even if he didn't, it wouldn't have been a problem. I met some cool blokes who are mates to this day. I was out of my comfort zone that's for sure. But I loved the experience and ended up going back for another two summers.

This trip down memory lane kind of reminds me how you might be feeling now. When you know you need to do something about the situation you're in now.

Grumpy.

Tired.

Clothes don't fit.

No energy.

Frustrated.

But also scared. Scared of the situation that you ended up in. But also scared of what needs to be done to change it.

You're nervous when you pluck up the courage to start. I get it, trust me. But stick it out and hang in there because it gets better.

It's just like my summer camp experience. You'll start to feel better. You'll have a little bit more energy each day and even start to find things a little easier during each workout.

You can even move a little better the next day after those first couple of workouts! That soreness is not as bad as what you expected. And hang on a minute, aren't those jeans feeling a little bit easier to slip on now?

Your friends are starting to notice how your face is looking slimmer. Your confidence seems to be returning and your partner starts paying you more attention.

Yes! It's happening! You're doing it! So take that first step. I guarantee you that it's worth it

New Miracle Drug

How good would it be if you could pop a pill or sip a drink that did the work for you? I mean losing the weight we wanted to lose, shrinking that flabby tummy and getting rid of the chunky thighs.

I'd get rid of my big butt and thighs that make me hate buying jeans. Definitely no skinny jeans for me!

But, back to this miracle drug thing. I once read an interview with a bloke called Adam Silver. He's the boss of the NBA. He'd met the top doctor in the United States, The Surgeon General. And he talked about this new drug that should take off. Well, it isn't really new.

According to Adam Silver, the Surgeon General is one of those people who are saying there's a miracle drug right now in this country. It's exercise.

Yep, good old-fashioned getting up and moving. Disappointing if you were waiting for that miracle pill right?

But seriously, that's all it takes. Just doing a little bit more than you're doing now.

And I don't necessarily mean joining a gym or joining DPM. It might just be playing with the kids more or it might just be walking around the block a few times.

Or it may well be the workouts in this book. That'll give you six months of action.

Whatever it is for you, just start something.

Trust The Process

Maybe you haven't exercised in months. Maybe even years. Or maybe the last time you did some exercise was when they called last drinks at the bar and you had to make a mad rush? Or chasing after your kids when they're about to sprint across a busy car park just to test you?

I know it can be intimidating when you start to think about exercise, or what it's often made out to be. You know the sweat soaked t-shirt and red face selfie that someone posts on Facebook or Instagram to 'inspire you' with the accompanying #fitspo. And every other hash tag that follows.

BUT, it doesn't have to be like that. You can start slowly. You can do half of a workout if that's all you have time for, or if that's all your body can initially take.

As long as you do something. I'm not going to lie and paint pictures of rainbows and unicorns, and angels singing as you get your body moving. It isn't a movie. Yes, your body will be a little sore. How sore?

Well that depends on whether you flog yourself or start smart. Start smart and you'll get a little bit of soreness in your body in the right spots to let you know that you did something. Flog yourself and you won't be able to get out of bed. That's not what I'm about.

But there's one thing I can guarantee you after you finish. You'll feel better pretty much straight away. Your brain will release some chemicals 'the feel good endorphins' to give you a kick.

So hang in there and trust the process. You'll feel mentally and physically better.

So, start with something and don't be intimated by what's ahead.

Take the plunge. You'll appreciate it in only four short weeks when you start to notice those pants getting easier to slide over your thighs. You'll even be able to slip into something you haven't been able to wear for a while. Then you'll be ready for the next workout.

Get Out Of Jail Free Card?

Let me take a wild stab in the dark. You enjoy a drink?

No shame there because I'll put my hand up here too. Both hands in fact! Give me a good red or a nice whisky. We'd get along quite well.

So if you do like a drink or three, here's some good news for you. Apart from helping to keep your sanity together, research shows that people who drink alcohol are less likely to die from cancer if they're physically active. Pretty cool right?

The findings were published in the British Journal of Sports Medicine. Researchers found physical activity might decrease the risks of dying from cancer and other illnesses.

Because if you're active, it's ok for you to enjoy a few drinks here and there.

Of course, the researchers did point out that it doesn't give you the license to drink more just because you exercise. But that's stating the obvious don't you think?

Ask anyone who's trying to lose weight if that holds up. Nope. But all in all, hearing this news is a good thing. Maybe even a little reassuring?

I'll tell you what gives you that bit of reassurance. Getting moving again. So, if you've got some damage to undo, use these workouts to get started and follow along at your own pace.

Just like you drink at your own pace, you can do the workouts at your own pace. Work at increasing your speed. It won't take you long until you're flying through them and getting more reps done in the same amount of time!

Frequently Asked Questions

Q: I'm not sure how to do some of the exercises. Do you have any demonstrations?

A: I describe how to do each exercise, including the warm-up ones, in the exercise library section of Short 'N Sweet that begins on page 37. There's also a video demo of every exercise on the download page for Short 'N Sweet at dpmworkout.com

Or invest in a DPM package and you'll get access to video links and an app so you can do the workouts with me in real-time at home.

Q: Why are some warm-ups and stretches only one minute long?

A: There's a simple answer. To keep the workouts to 20 minutes as advertised. Sure, if you have time, take longer. But too many trainers advertise programs that only take XYZ minutes but forget to mention the warm-up and stretches.

This isn't going to be dangerous for you because it's not as if you're warming up for a minute then going straight into lifting your maximum weight at the gym. Your body will continue to warm up as you do the workout.

Q: What if the workouts are too hard?

A: There's a written description of the beginner and advanced versions for each exercise in the exercise library that begins on page 37. The video demonstrations will also show you how you can scale things back if it is too hard for you. Just increase when your body is ready for it.

Q: What if the workouts are too easy?

A: Same as above but in reverse. Step things up by following the advanced exercise examples. You can also use things like bands and rollers to make the exercises harder to do.

If it's still too easy, don't use the rest period. Do an in-betweener exercise like Reverse Helicopters, Leg Shuffles, Stick Ups or even Shadow Boxing instead of the downtime/transition period.

Q: What if I can't complete a workout or an exercise for a certain timer duration?

A: Do what you can. Rest when you need to and build from there. Keep the timer ticking and aim to reduce your overall rest time. You'll be surprised by how quickly you can improve.

The most important thing is to do what's right for your situation right now. If you haven't exercised in a while, err on the side of caution and see how your body pulls up the next day.

A little bit of muscle soreness is okay. If you can't get out of bed, you've obviously pushed yourself too hard. I'd much rather you ease in and do more the next time.

Q: I don't have enough time for a full workout. Is it even worth it and what should I do?

A: Yes of course. Doing anything is better than doing nothing. I guarantee you'll benefit from even a five or ten minute workout. Your body and brain will benefit. And you'll feel good because you did something.

No matter how 'little' you may think it is. Remember it all adds up. Customise the number of sets you do for the time you have available.

Q: I've got an injury or problem areas that stop me from doing certain exercises. What should I do?

A: There are lots of different options in the exercise library section of this book and in the video demonstrations that I can share with you.

Of course, first make sure you speak with your doctor about your condition and whether it's appropriate to start.

Q: How long should I stick with each workout for?

A: These workouts are designed to be followed for one month each. Once you've completed the first month, move on to month two and so on until you've completed them all.

Q: How many times a week should I do each workout?

A: To be honest, anything is better than doing nothing as you may have guessed by reading some of the earlier bits of this book. But ideally, you want to try to aim for three workouts each week if you're looking to lose weight or two if you want to maintain where you are currently.

Remember, you don't need to commit heaps of time. 20 minutes maximum. So that should be doable right? But remember, even once or twice a week will still help. It'll just take longer to notice the benefits.

Q: Do you have a template or something I can use to track my workouts each month?

A: You'll find one for each workout on the resources page at dpmworkout.com in both excel and pdf format.

Have I missed anything?

Email me at daniel@dpmtransformation.com and I'll do my best to answer your question.

Workout Explanations

The six workouts all use a timer. So you're guaranteed the workouts will take a maximum of 20 minutes.

Now, I'll reiterate that if you are a beginner, and not used to regular exercise, get a clearance from your doctor before you start. Take this book with you to show them what you're planning to begin and make sure that it's appropriate for your current situation.

Same goes if you have injury concerns that may prevent you from doing particular exercises. Pick an alternative that you'll find in the exercise library that doesn't compromise your injury history.

Remember, if you're not sure about what to do after watching the exercise video demonstrations or the follow along with me workout (that you can invest in at dpmworkout.com), then ask a qualified trainer to show you how to do the exercises properly so you don't hurt yourself.

The other important thing to remember is to work at your own pace even though you're using a timer for the workouts. Don't do too much for your body. The last thing you need is to push yourself too hard, so that you end up not being able to move or sit down the next day. Or even worse, injure yourself because you went too hard, too soon.

It's no shame to admit that neither of us are 21 anymore right! So work at your pace. Sit out if you need to get your breath back. Sit out half of a round and resume when you're able. Build up slowly. Because every single workout counts. No matter how little or how much of it you actually do.

Remember, half a workout is better than no workout right? And to be honest, you'll be surprised at how quickly your body will adapt and have you able to be doing more.

And if you have more questions, just send me an email at daniel@dpmtransformation.com and I'll do my best to help you.

MONTH 1: New Beginnings

WARM UP ROUTINE - 2 MINS
- Chest Press x 10
- Spiderman Twists x 10
- Squats x 10
- Waiters Bow x 10

Repeat as many times as possible for 2 minutes. If you're a beginner, rest when needed.

TIMER SUPERSETS:
The idea here is to work on a 20/10 timer ratio. That means 20 seconds of work and 10 seconds of rest for each exercise. Repeat each superset (e.g. 1a and 1b for 4 times, which equals 4 minutes).

If you can't complete the full 20 seconds without stopping, keep the timer running but have a quick break, reset and resume.

Work up to eventually being able to go through without pausing until you reach the 10-second rest period.

1a) Push Ups x 20 seconds with 10 seconds rest before next exercise
1b) Hamstring Lifts x 20 seconds with 10 seconds rest
Repeat x 4 rounds for 4 minutes total

2a) Stick Ups x 20 seconds with 10 seconds rest before next exercise
2b) Prisoner Squats x 20 seconds with 10 seconds rest
Repeat x 4 rounds for 4 minutes total

3a) Step Body Blasts x 20 seconds with 10 seconds rest before next exercise
3b) Leg Shuffles x 20 seconds with 10 seconds rest
Repeat x 4 rounds for 4 minutes total

4a) Side Plank Pumps Left Side x 20 seconds with 10 seconds rest before next exercise
4b) Side Plank Pumps Right Side x 20 seconds with 10 seconds rest
Repeat x 4 rounds for 4 minutes total

STRETCH - 2 MINS (follow video on the download page or your own).

NOTE: If you have time, you can stretch for longer, and I recommend you do. This is a very brief stretch, but anything is better than nothing.

DPM Success Story: Ginny - Busy Mum & Grandmother

"Before I started this program I was feeling pretty lethargic and uncomfortable in a lot of my clothes. I knew I had to do something to get back in shape and feel better about myself.

Now I feel much better about myself and see the progress I am making on my journey to fitness! One of the biggest changes for me is that I now get up early and do my workouts. Then it is done and anything else I do is extra!

If I don't make myself get up and workout I feel out of sorts during the day. I also find that I am more tired if I do not workout so it's true that I have more energy!

I have tried many other plans such as Weight Watchers, Atkins, South Beach and I've done the Whole 30. I like the ease of doing your plan and I can fit it into my schedule.

I have lost weight and inches and I will continue to lose more! I had gotten pretty lazy before I started this plan, but now I realise that the hardest part is just starting. I see that the choice is totally up to me! And that I am capable of my own fitness journey and can keep going.

I would tell someone considering this plan to just start! Small steps can make a big difference in attitude. It is a lifestyle change, but it is practical and doable.

I feel so much better about my choices than I did four weeks ago! I know I can continue to progress and maintain my goals. Thank You Daniel"

- Ginny, busy mum and grandmother in the USA who followed the DPM 4 Week Online Program.

MONTH 2: The Next Episode

WARM UP ROUTINE – 2 MINS
- T Squats x 10
- Hover Hold x 10 secs
- Push Ups x 10 (knees are fine)
- Split Squats x 10 each leg

Repeat as many times as possible for 2 minutes. If you're a beginner, rest when needed.

TIMER CIRCUIT
The idea here is to work on a 40/20 timer ratio. That means 40 seconds of work and 20 seconds of rest for each exercise before moving on to the next one in the circuit. Once you've completed it all once, repeat again (for 2 sets total).

If you can't complete the full 40 seconds without stopping, keep the timer running but have a quick break, reset and resume.

Work up to eventually being able to go through without pausing until you reach the 20-second rest period.

1. One Arm Hover Holds Left Arm x 40 seconds work, 20 seconds rest
2. One Arm Hover Holds Right Arm x 40 seconds work, 20 seconds rest
3. Backstrokers x 40 seconds work, 20 seconds rest
4. Waves x 40 seconds work, 20 seconds rest
5. Figure 4's Left Leg x 40 seconds work, 20 seconds rest
6. Figure 4's Right Leg x 40 seconds work, 20 seconds rest
7. Stick Ups with Calf Raises x 40 seconds work, 20 seconds rest
8. Crossover Star Jumps x 40 seconds work, 20 seconds rest
Repeat x 2 sets total

STRETCH - 2 MINS (follow video on the download page or do your own).

NOTE: If you have time, you can stretch for longer, and I recommend you do. This is a very brief stretch through in the two minutes, but as always, anything is better than nothing.

DPM Success Story: Kate - Busy Mum Of Three

Q: How did you feel before you started your online training with me?

A: I felt bloated. I knew I had to do something but couldn't do it alone. I need the support and someone to encourage and keep me on track.

Q: What are the biggest differences that you've noticed one month in?

A: I feel lighter. I haven't lost a lot of weight but looking back on my before and after pictures, I can see the difference. The scales might not show much but I know I achieved something!! I can feel it!

Q: How do you feel about yourself now?

A: Last time I did this I was going to Fiji. I remember the confidence I had walking around the pool in a bikini. I wanted that again.

I wanted to show my four-year-old daughter what a confident mum of three should look like.

Q: What stopped you from starting sooner?

A: Scared of failing. I have tried it before on my own, but I noticed myself having that one glass of wine (no one will know). I know I can't do it alone!

Q: What have you tried before, if anything?

A: I have done the DPM 28 day challenge two years ago almost! It worked! I wouldn't even bother trying anything else. This is easy when I'm motivated!

Exercises are easy. The food plan is easy to follow. No tricky recipes or ingredients you haven't heard of before! Simple and easy!!

Q: What would you say to someone who may be in the exact spot you were four weeks ago?

A: It's easy! If it's support you need Daniel is the right person to help you! He will support, encourage, and motivate you! It's honestly the easiest 28-day challenge.

Even after the 28 days, the exercise and food intake becomes part of your life.

For lunch the other day I had steamed broccoli and pumpkin with chilli flakes. I didn't know how much I'd enjoy this type of food. I liked eggs and avocado for breakfast! That's just normal for me now.

Thank you, thank you, thank you Daniel!!

MONTH 3: Shadow Boxer

WARM UP ROUTINE – 1 MIN
- Squats x 10
- Waiters Bow x 10
- Spiderman Twists x 10

Repeat as many times as possible for 1 minute. If you're a beginner, rest when needed.

TIMER SUPERSETS
The idea here is to work on a 45/15 timer ratio. That means 45 seconds of work and 15 seconds of rest for each exercise before moving on to the next one. Once you've completed it all once, repeat again twice (for three sets total).

If you can't complete the full 45 seconds without stopping, keep the timer running but have a quick break, reset and resume.

Work up to eventually being able to go through until the 15-second rest period.

1a) Left-Left-Right punches at Chest Height x 45 seconds work, with 15 seconds rest before next exercise
1b) Right-Right-Left punches at Chest Height x 45 seconds work, with 15 seconds rest
Repeat x 3 sets

2a) Left Jabs at Chest Height x 45 seconds work, with 15 seconds rest before next exercise
2b) Right Jabs at Chest Height x 45 seconds work, with 15 seconds rest
Repeat x 3 sets

3a) Double Punches at Chest Height HARD x 45 seconds work, with 15 seconds rest before next exercise
3b) Jump Backs x 45 seconds work, with 15 seconds rest
Repeat x 3 sets

STRETCH - 1 MIN (follow video on the download page or do your own).

NOTE: If you have time, stretch for longer of course, but this will help.

DPM Success Story: Melinda - Busy Mum Of Two

Ever felt that it's all too hard to start making some small changes? Sure, sometimes it is. But if you break things down it can become pretty simple. Here's an example straight from the DPM Success Files.

Melinda is a busy mum. She works and has a family. A pretty full-on schedule I'm sure you'd agree. Just like yours. But over three months she did something amazing.

And truth be told, I haven't even met Melinda in person. She did it all remotely without a face-to-face session. Just like you can too by following this book.

The weight loss on the scales was impressive (7.5kg). But the real change, as per usual, was the measurement change. VERY significant.

* 5.5 cm from around her belly button

* 6 cm from her hips

* 5.5 cm off her thighs

I could go on, but rather than continue to throw these numbers at you, I questioned Melinda to find out what her secret was (apart from the DPM programming of course!)

There are some cool insights here, which may help you with your own challenge.

Q: How did you feel before you started your online training with me?

A: I felt tired, lethargic and chubby before I started the online training. I really needed something to turn my life around.

Q: What are the biggest differences that you've noticed three months in?

A: The biggest difference that I've noticed in the last three months is the loss of weight. I feel more fit and more energetic.

Q: How do you feel about yourself now?

A: I feel happy within myself and know I'm doing the right thing for my body as well as the right thing for my kids. I want to live a long, healthy and happy life for my kids.

Q: What stopped you from starting sooner?

A: I didn't want to go to a gym and had never found a program that motivated me. The online training motivated me because I could do the training in the comfort of my own home with no strangers spectating and I can do it at a time that suits me.

Also having you check-in on my progress every week motivates me to keep on top of my workouts.

Q: What have you tried before, if anything?

A: I've tried going to the gym before (that didn't end well, only in major embarrassment) and have done yoga classes.

But classes don't fit into my busy schedule as a mum these days as they don't hold them late at night after the kids have gone to bed.

Q: What would you say to someone who may be in the exact spot you were three months ago?

A: I would say give it a go. You never know unless you try. I'm a pretty lazy person so if I can do it and stick to it then anyone can.

Melinda's story, and the others shared in this book, proves that you don't have to dedicate hours each day to the cause. Just follow the plan and implement what you discover in this book because it works!

MONTH 4: Circuit Special

WARM UP ROUTINE – 2 MINS
* Stick Ups with Calf Raises x 10
* Hover Hold x 10 secs
* Double Punches at Chest Height x 10
* Split Squats x 10 each leg

Repeat as many times as possible for 2 minutes. If you're a beginner, rest when needed.

TIMER CIRCUIT
The idea here is to work on a 30/30 timer ratio. That means 30 seconds of work and straight into 30 seconds of the next exercise in the circuit without any rest. Once you've completed it all once, repeat the circuit twice more (for three sets total).

If you can't complete the full 30 seconds without stopping, keep the timer running but have a quick break, reset and resume.

Work up to eventually being able to go through without pausing until you finish all three complete sets.

1. Wall Sit x 30 seconds hold
2. Monster Walks x 30 seconds (two steps forward, two steps back)
3. Step Leg Shuffles x 30 seconds
4. Jump Backs x 30 seconds
5. V Sit Hold x 30 seconds
6. Up & Overs x 30 seconds
7. Diamond Push Ups x 30 seconds
8. Reverse Helicopters x 30 seconds
Repeat x 3 sets total

(OPTION: Do 4 sets if that's easy and you have the time, this will take 20 minutes total workout time)

STRETCH - 2 MINS (follow video on the download page or do your own).

NOTE: If you have time, you can stretch for longer, and I recommend you do. This is a very brief stretch through in the two minutes, but as always, anything is better than nothing.

DPM Success Story: Kasey - Busy Mum Of Two

Q: How did you feel before you started this program with me?

A: Was feeling bloated, unmotivated, low energy and just "blurghhh". My clothes were tighter and I was eating more junk food than usual.

Q: What are the biggest differences that you've noticed four weeks in?

A: Increased energy (huge), more focused, less bloated, happier, mentally sharper and overall just feel better. I don't crave salty or sweet food as much either.

Q: How do you feel about yourself now?

A: Proud that I have made these changes. I'm no longer reaching for the pretzels and wine when I walk in the door at night. I feel less moody, happier and clothes are fitting better too.

Q: What stopped you from starting sooner?

A: Lack of motivation and had no accountability. I had gotten into a rut and found it hard to get out. I had all the tools - cookbook, knowledge etc. but lacked the drive to make the change.

Q: What have you tried before, if anything?

A: I didn't try anything. I'd looked at a healthy gut diet but didn't start it.

Q: What would you say to someone who may be in the exact spot you were only four short weeks ago?

A: I'd say that four weeks is such a short time to make such a huge change. I would encourage anyone to do this four-week course and to do it at least once a year to re-adjust any bad habits. I loved the challenges.

MONTH 5: Combo Crazies

WARM UP ROUTINE – 1 MIN
* Squat and Drive x 10
* Stick Ups x 10
* Spiderman Twists x 10

Repeat as many times as possible for 1 minute. If you're a beginner, rest when needed.

SHADOW BOXING BODYWEIGHT TIMER CIRCUIT
The idea here is to work on a 60/60 timer ratio. That means 60 seconds of work and straight into 60 seconds of the next exercise in the circuit without any rest. Once you've completed it all once, repeat again (for two sets total).

If you can't complete the full 60 seconds without stopping, keep the timer running but have a quick break, reset and resume.

Work up to eventually being able to go through without pausing until you finish both complete sets.

1. Left-Right Punches at Chest Height - Slow and Hard x 60 seconds
2. Sprinters Shuffles x 60 seconds
3. Forearm Walks x 60 seconds
4. Single Leg Hip Extensions Left Leg x 60 seconds
5. Single Leg Hip Extensions Right Leg x 60 seconds
6. One Arm Hover Extensions Left Arm x 60 seconds
7. One Arm Hover Extensions Right Arm x 60 seconds
8. Ski Jumps x 60 seconds
9. Double Punches at Chest Height - Fast x 60 seconds
Repeat x 2 sets total

STRETCH - 1 MIN (follow video on the download page or do your own.)

NOTE: If you have time, you can stretch for longer, and I recommend you do. This is a very brief stretch through (especially in one minute), but as always, anything is better than nothing.

DPM Success Story: David - Busy Dad Of Three (Yes, It Even Works For Blokes!)

Q: How did you feel before you started this program with me?

A: I felt lost as to how I was going to build on my fitness program. I was stagnant and couldn't get under 88kg.

Q: What are the biggest differences that you've noticed four weeks in?

A: The lower bloat I have.

Q: How do you feel about yourself now?

A: That I can do better still. Have even lost more in the last week after a huge weekend bender.

Q: What stopped you from starting sooner?

A: I didn't know who to talk to.

Q: What have you tried before, if anything?

A: Just fitness and eating well. But lots of carbs and dairy.

Q: What would you say to someone who may be in the exact spot you were only four short weeks ago?

A: Have a crack. Heaps of protein, green veggies, no carbs, and no milk.

I needed help to break the floor. I will continue with the diet massively. My body rejects bad food now. It's crazy.

MONTH 6: Aim Up

WARM UP ROUTINE – 2 MINS
* Stick Ups x 10
* Waiters Bows x 10
* Reverse Helicopters x 10
* Prisoner Squats x 10

Repeat as many times as possible for 2 minutes. If you're a beginner, rest when needed.

CARDIO ABS TIMER SUPERSETS:

The game plan here is another 20/10 timer ratio like you did back in month one. As per usual, aim to get all the way through the 20 seconds before resting but if you need to stop, minimise the down time.

1a) Spiderman Twists x 20 seconds with 10 seconds rest before next exercise
1b) Virtual Skipping x 20 seconds with 10 seconds rest
Repeat x 4 rounds for 4 minutes total

2a) Hand Walks x 20 seconds with 10 seconds rest before next exercise
2b) Scissor Squats x 20 seconds with 10 seconds rest before next exercise
Repeat x 4 rounds for 4 minutes total

3a) One Arm Hover Holds Left Arm x 20 seconds with 10 seconds rest before next exercise
3b) One Arm Hover Holds Right Arm x 20 seconds with 10 seconds rest
Repeat x 4 rounds for 4 minutes total

4a) Leg Blaster Left Leg x 20 seconds with 10 seconds rest before next exercise
4b) Leg Blaster Right Leg x 20 seconds with 10 seconds rest
Repeat x 4 rounds for 4 minutes total

STRETCH - 2 MINS (follow video on the download page or do your own.)

NOTE: If you have time, you can stretch for longer, and I recommend you do. This is a very brief stretch through (especially in one minute), but as always, anything is better than nothing.

DPM Success Story: Jessica - Busy Mum Of Three

Q: How do you feel about yourself now?

A: Happier. More confident. Pleased my clothes fit. Inspired to lose 3kg!

Q: What stopped you from starting sooner?

A: I got into a rut after eating throughout my pregnancy. Also had to wait until I got the green light to exercise again from the doctors after having a baby.

Q: What have you tried before, if anything?

A: Exercise and diets, but I've never keep it up.

Q: What would you say to someone who may be in the exact spot you were only four short weeks ago?

A: Get yourself moving and eating better. You will be surprised by the results in just four short weeks and it will inspire you to do more!

Exercise Library

Here's a list of every single exercise (in alphabetical order) that's in this book. The warm-up exercises are included too.

I describe how to do each exercise in simple terms. Plus, I indicate which part/s of the body the exercises are working. You can also check out the video demonstrations on the DPM Resources page here:

dpmworkout.com

Backstrokers
1. Sit on the ground with your knees bent.
2. Place your hands by your sides on the ground (what way they face is up to you - I prefer hands facing forward) and lift your hips up.
3. Hold your hips off the ground so your thighs are as close to parallel to the ground as possible. (How high you can lift your hips depends on your flexibility).
4. Kick one leg out in front of you so it goes no higher than your thigh height and alternate with the other leg.

- Where should you feel it?
The back of your legs (hamstrings), butt (glutes), triceps (back of your arms) and the higher you lift your thighs the more you'll feel it in your quads (front of thighs) and your abs too.

Bulgarian Split Squats
1. Place your back leg on a lounge or a chair. Your front leg will be in front of your body at a comfortable stance with your foot pointing straight ahead.
2. Bend your front knee making sure that all the weight of that front leg is driving down through your front heel. You don't want your knee going forward over your toes.
3. Your back leg will move down when you bend your front leg and lower as far as you can before raising and repeating.
4. Elevating your back leg increases the intensity of a normal Split Squat. Hold on to something if you can't keep your balance. Try to look at something straight ahead or put your finger in your belly button to help you balance (this sounds silly but it works surprisingly well).

- Where should you feel it?
When you drive down through your front heel, you'll feel it work deeper in the front of your back thigh (quads) and in your front leg you'll feel your hamstrings (back of the leg) and your glutes (butt.)

Crossover Star Jumps

1. Stand as you would to do a regular Star Jump with your feet just outside shoulder width and your arms by your side.
2. Jump your legs apart as far as you can comfortably go while at the same time extending your arms out so they are parallel to the ground.
3. Bring your legs in to the start position while at the same time crossing your arms in front of your chest so that your hands are stretched out on the opposite side of your body.

- Where should you feel it?
This is a cardio exercise that's great for getting your heart rate up. You may feel your inner thighs from jumping your legs in and out, and your shoulders and arms from the crossover movement, but they're not the primary target.

Diamond Push Ups

1. This exercise is similar to a regular push up but harder to do. Beginners start on their knees. The degree of intensity increases the further your thighs are leaning forward away from your knees. This just means that your starting position for your hands is further away from your knees. Keep increasing the intensity until you are ready to move to your toes.
2. Or start on your toes. But only do this if you can keep your body in a straight line without your hips sagging at the bottom of the movement.
3. Your hands will be placed in a diamond position just under your chest. The tips of your thumb and index finger on each hand should be touching or as close together as possible.
4. Lower your body down towards the ground. The lower you go the harder it is. Make sure your elbows are brushing your sides as you lower towards the ground.
5. When you're as low as possible, ideally your chest is just above the ground, come back up to the beginning position and repeat for the desired number of repetitions.

- Where should you feel it?
Primarily your triceps (backs of your arms) and your chest and shoulders (deltoids.)

Double Punches at Chest Height

1. For this punching combo you're best to stand in a neutral position (feet just outside shoulder width apart like you're doing a Squat) instead of your traditional boxing stance.
2. Place your arms at chest height and close your fists as if you're

punching.

3. Quickly push your arms in and out as if you are punching a target at chest height.
4. The difference with these punches is you are throwing both hands at the same time instead of your usual 1-2 combination.

- Where should you feel it?

Your lats (back muscles), chest, shoulders and triceps (backs of your arms.) Your abs will also work as you are standing in a neutral position and you can notice a cardio benefit from your heart rate increasing.

Figure 4's
1. Lay on your back with one knee bent with that foot flat on the ground.
2. Your other leg is going to make a figure 4 (hence the name of the exercise) by resting that ankle on the bent knee of the leg on the ground.
3. Lift your hips up as high as your flexibility allows and lower towards the ground making sure your butt stays off the ground with each repetition.
4. Swap legs once you've completed the desired number of repetitions.

- Where should you feel it?

The figure 4 makes sure your glutes (butt) work on both legs. You'll also notice your hamstrings (back of upper leg) and your inner thigh on your leg making the 4.

Forearm Walks
1. Begin in a hover position with your forearms on the ground with your elbows under your shoulders and your knees on the ground. The degree of intensity increases the further your thighs are leaning forward away from your knees.
2. Move one forearm out in front of your body about 3-5cm and bring the other one out to meet it. Repeat the process walking in the first forearm then the second until you're in the starting position again.
3. That counts as one repetition. Repeat for as long as necessary.
4. If you're a beginner, start on your knees with your thighs and your lower leg in a 90-degree angle, and work your thighs forwards from there if that becomes easy.
5. NOTE: You may need a towel or padding under your elbows so you don't graze them. If that still doesn't work, do a hand walk (mentioned below) instead.

- Where should you feel it?

Primarily in your abs and obliques in the sides of your midsection. You'll also feel your shoulders and arms work. It's also a great cardio exercise as it can be quite intense which means you're working harder!

Hamstring Lifts

1. Lie on your back and place both feet elevated on a chair or a lounge (the further you're away from that object the harder it will be).
2. To make it harder, place your heels on the highest point possible. To make it easier, place the soles of your feet against the side of the lounge so your whole foot is covered. This takes out some of the intensity.
3. Lift your hips in the air as high as your flexibility allows. Make sure you squeeze your butt when you get towards the top of the movement.
4. Lower and repeat for the desired number of repetitions making sure your butt stays off the ground each time.

- Where should you feel it?

Your hamstrings in the back of your legs and your butt. The higher you lift your hips the more you will likely feel it in the front of your thighs (quads) and your abs.

Hand Walks

1. Begin in a push-up position with your hands on the ground under your shoulders. Hold your body up on your toes so your back is parallel to the ground.
2. Move one hand out in front of your body about 3-5cm and bring the other one out to meet it. Repeat the process walking in the first hand then the second until you're in the starting position again.
3. Repeat for as many repetitions as necessary.
4. If you're a beginner, you will need to do this on your knees as you would for a push-up on your knees.

- Where should you feel it?

Primarily in your abs and obliques in the sides of your midsection. You'll also feel your shoulders and arms work. It's also a great cardio exercise as it can be quite intense which means you're working harder!

Jump Backs

1. Stand with your feet shoulder width apart.
2. Jump both feet back together about 5 cm or so making sure you are landing on the balls of your feet. You don't want to over exaggerate this movement and land with a thud. That'll place too much stress on your back and joints.
3. Repeat that motion, jumping forwards and landing on the balls of your feet again for as many repetitions as necessary.

4. Back then forwards counts as two in your count.

- Where should you feel it?

This is purely a cardio exercise designed to get your heart rate up in limited space. Your calf muscles (backs of your lower legs) may feel it a little bit too.

Left-Left-Right at Chest Height - Slow and Hard
1. Hold your hands in front of your chin in a boxing stance. Your left foot will be standing forward for this version, with your left closed fist slightly in front of the right closed fist. Your thumbs will be facing closest towards your body.
2. Punch out as if you're hitting a boxing bag or focus pads. Make sure you turn your hand so your closed palm is facing the ground and your knuckles are facing the roof.
3. Pull your punch back when your arm is almost completely extended so the speed of the movement is mimicking a slow and hard punching action.
4. Repeat that for your left arm, quickly followed by a hard right punch going across your body making sure you turn your hips towards the punch as you are performing the motion.
5. This left, left, right punch combo counts as one repetition in your total count and repeat for the desired number of repetitions.

- Where should you feel it?

Boxing can become a total body workout when you turn your hip into the punch that goes across the body. You'll feel both arms (primarily the left arm in this combo), your shoulders, the lat muscles that run down each side of your back and your abs. Your back leg will also get some action when you're turning your hip towards the right punch.

Left-Right Punches at Chest Height - Slow and Hard
1. Hold your hands in front of your chin in a boxing stance. Your left foot will be standing forward for this version, with your left closed fist slightly in front of the right closed fist. Your thumbs will be facing closest towards your body.
2. Punch out as if you're hitting a boxing bag or focus pads. Make sure you turn your hand so your closed palm is facing the ground and your knuckles are facing the roof.
3. Pull your punch back when your arm is almost completely extended so the speed of the movement is mimicking a slow and hard punching action.
4. Follow that punch with a hard right punch going across your body making sure you turn your hips towards the punch as you are performing the motion.
5. Count each punch individually towards your total count with this

combination and repeat for the desired number of repetitions.

- Where should you feel it?
Boxing can become a total body workout when you turn your hip into the punch that goes across the body. You'll feel both arms, your shoulders, the lat muscles that run down each side of your back and your abs. Your back leg will also get some action when you are turning your hip towards the right punch.

Left Jabs at Chest Height - Fast
1. Hold your hands in front of your chin in a boxing stance. Your left foot will be standing forward for this version, with your left closed fist slightly in front of the right closed fist. Your thumbs will be facing closest towards your body.
2. Punch out as if you're hitting a boxing bag or focus pads. Make sure you turn your hand so your closed palm is facing the ground and your knuckles are facing the roof.
3. Quickly pull your punch back when your arm is almost completely extended so the speed of the movement is mimicking a fast punching action and repeat for the desired number of repetitions.

- Where should you feel it?
Your left arm will definitely be working as will the left shoulder. The beauty of shadow boxing is your lats in your back and your obliques and abs will be working too, this time on your left side. It's a lot more effective than it looks!

Leg Blaster
1. Lie on your back with one knee bent and that foot flat on the ground.
2. Raise your other leg so that it's perpendicular to the floor or at a position that's comfortable for your flexibility.
3. Lift your hips up in the air so your butt comes off the ground and you're lifting your hips as high as your flexibility allows.
4. As you're raising your hips, stand up on your toes so that your heel is elevated off the ground and lower your heel and your hips to complete the movement.
5. Squeeze your butt when you get toward the top of the movement to make the glutes work a bit harder.
6. Make sure your butt stays off the ground on the way back down, stopping just above the floor. Repeat for the desired number of repetitions then do the same on the other leg.

- Where should you feel it?
Pretty much everywhere in your leg that's working. You should feel your hamstrings in the back of your leg and your glutes (butt) as you are

raising your hips. You should also feel your calf muscle when you rise up onto your toes.

Leg Shuffles
1. Stand with your feet about shoulder width apart.
2. Keep your weight on the balls of your feet and shift your legs back and forwards like you're moving your feet in a scissor movement.
3. Back and forwards counts as two repetitions in this instance.

- Where should you feel it?
This is purely a great cardio exercise designed to get your heart rate up.

Monster Walks
1. Stand as you would for a normal Squat with your feet just outside shoulder width apart.
2. Squat down and hold that position as low as you can comfortably go. Make sure your knees aren't over your toes and that all your weight is going back through your heels. Try to imagine you have to sit back on a chair that's further away than you expected.
3. While you're holding this position walk one leg backwards about 3-5cm.
4. Bring your other leg back past the first leg so you are walking backwards in a staggered motion.
5. Go straight into the two forward steps, coming back to the starting position and alternating for the timer duration between backwards and forwards.

- Where should you feel it?
Mainly in the front of your thighs (quads) and the backs of your legs (hamstrings) and butt as you would for a normal Squat hold. The extra benefit here is your butt and inner thighs will work harder especially when walking backwards.

One Arm Hover Extensions
1. Assume a hover (plank) position with your forearms on the ground.
2. Beginners will want to be on their knees. (The greater the angle of your thighs leaning forward, the harder the intensity.) More advanced people will be on their toes.
3. Extend one arm in front of your body, resting on just the one forearm (and supporting your body on your toes/knees).
4. Bring that arm back to the body and repeat extending the same arm in and out for the prescribed number of repetitions.
5. Repeat the same on the other side.

- Where should you feel it?

In your abs down the front of your tummy. You'll also feel it in your obliques (sides of the midsection) on the side that's extending in and out and on the side holding your body on the ground. You may feel it in the shoulder of your grounded arm and in the front of the arm on the side you're extending.

One Arm Hover Holds

1. As per the above example with one forearm resting on the ground and you're holding yourself up by your toes. Choose the knee option if you're a beginner.
2. The difference is you're holding an arm out in front of you without bringing it back in for the desired time.

- Where should you feel it?

Same as above. In your abs, obliques, shoulder on the ground and arm raised out in front of your body.

Prisoner Squats

1. Stand in a regular Squat position with your feet just outside shoulder width apart.
2. Place your hands behind your head, interlocking your fingers as if you are a prisoner (hence the name.)
3. Squat as per normal by lowering your butt towards the ground as low as you can comfortably go. For most people this is just above your thighs being parallel to the ground.
4. Stand up to your beginning position making sure your hands stay behind your head the whole time.
5. When your hands are in the prisoner position, your knees will want to go forward as you squat. To avoid this, place all your weight through your heels as you sit back and push your butt back as if you're sitting down on a chair that's further behind you than expected.

- Where should you feel it?

As you would normally for a regular Squat, in the front and back of your thighs (quads and hamstrings) and your glutes. The upper body gets a workout here too with the prisoner movement meaning your shoulders, trapezius (upper back muscles below your neck) are going to work too.

Push Ups

1. Two versions here, with beginners on your knees. The degree of intensity increases the further your thighs are leaning forward away from your knees. This just means that your starting position for your

hands is further away from your knees. Keep increasing the intensity until you are ready to move to your toes.
2. Or start on your toes. But only do this if you can keep your body in a straight line without your hips sagging at the bottom of the movement.
3. Your hands will be placed close to your shoulders just outside your chest.
4. Lower your body down towards the ground. The lower you go the harder it is. Make sure your elbows are brushing your sides as you lower towards the ground.
5. NOTE: A traditional push-up has your elbows flaring out as you lower the body. You can do this, but I like the elbows back version especially if you've had an elbow injury.
6. When you're as low as possible, ideally your chest is just above the ground, come back up to the beginning position and repeat for the desired number of repetitions.

- Where should you feel it?

Primarily your pecs in the front of your chest, your triceps in the backs of your arms and your shoulders (deltoids). Your abs will also work if you're doing this properly. When you start doing these with your feet elevated, or with your feet on a foam roller, you'll also work your lat muscles that run down the sides of your upper back.

Reverse Helicopters
1. Stand with your feet just outside shoulder width apart and with your arms elevated so that your arms are parallel to the ground.
2. Slowly rotate your arms in a backwards direction so that you are making small circles.
3. Don't over-exaggerate your circle motions. Smaller, shallower movements are better.
4. Repeat for the desired number of repetitions moving only in an anti-clockwise (backwards) direction.

- Where should you feel it?

This is a great exercise for working the small muscles in the backs of your shoulders (rear deltoid muscles and external rotator cuff muscles). You should also feel these in your upper back (trapezius muscles) at the base of your neck. I also find these are great to do if you're experiencing neck pain as they can sometimes help relieve your symptoms.

Right Jabs at Chest Height - Fast
1. Hold your hands in front of your chin in a boxing stance. Your right foot will be standing forward for this version, with your right closed

fist slightly in front of the left closed fist. Your thumbs will be facing closest towards your body.
2. Punch out as if you are hitting a boxing bag or focus pads. Make sure you turn your hand so your closed palm is facing the ground and your knuckles are facing the roof.
3. Quickly pull your punch back when your arm is almost completely extended so the speed of the movement is mimicking a fast punching action and repeat for the desired number of repetitions.

- Where should you feel it?
Your right arm will definitely be working as will the right shoulder. The beauty of shadow boxing is your lats in your back and your obliques and abs will be working too, this time on your right side.

Right-Right-Left at Chest Height - Slow and Hard
1. Hold your hands in front of your chin in a boxing stance. Your right foot will be standing forward for this version, with your right closed fist slightly in front of the left closed fist. Your thumbs will be facing closest towards your body.
2. Punch out as if you are hitting a boxing bag or focus pads. Make sure you turn your hand so your closed palm is facing the ground and your knuckles are facing the roof.
3. Pull your punch back when your arm is almost completely extended so the speed of the movement is mimicking a slow and hard punching action.
4. Repeat that for your right arm, quickly followed by a hard left punch going across your body making sure you turn your hips towards the punch as you are performing the motion.
5. This right, right, left punch combo counts as one repetition in your total count and repeat for the desired number of repetitions.

- Where should you feel it?
Boxing can become a total body workout when you turn your hip into the punch that goes across the body. You'll feel both arms (primarily the right arm in this combo), your shoulders, the lat muscles that run down each side of your back and your abs. Your back leg will also get some action when you are turning your hip towards the right punch.

Scissor Squats
1. Start in a regular Squat position with your feet just outside shoulder width apart.
2. As you are lowering your butt, jump your legs apart so when you land at the bottom of the Squat position your legs are as far apart as they can comfortably go.
3. Make sure when you do this motion you are sitting back as you would for a normal Squat so that your knees aren't extended over

your toes.
4. Return to the beginning position by jumping your legs back to their starting position as you are standing up from your squat position.
- Where should you feel it?

Same areas as a normal Squat. The addition here is your inner thighs. It also becomes a cardio exercise because it's more intense than a normal squat and gets your heart rate up.

Side Plank Pumps

1. You can start on your forearm or on your hand. The choice is up to you. The forearm will give you a greater base of support making it slightly easier to perform.
2. If you choose your forearm, make sure your shoulder is in line with your elbow. If you choose your hand, make sure your shoulder is in line with your wrist.
3. Use your forearm or hand to hold one side with your body off the floor. Position your feet how you like. Some people place the top leg on top of the bottom leg. I prefer placing the top leg slightly in front of the bottom leg on the ground. Some people find this gives you a little bit more stability.
4. If you're a beginner, you may need to rest your legs on the ground rather than relying on your body to hold you off the ground.
5. Raise your top arm above your head so it's pointing straight up to the roof. This is the normal Side Plank Hold position.
6. The Pump comes into it when you dip your hips down towards the floor (without touching the ground) and back up again for the desired number of repetitions. Then swap to the other side.
7. NOTE: If you have wrist or hand issues, only do this on your forearms.

- Where should you feel it?

Your oblique muscles in your midsection on the side facing the floor. The shoulder and arm of that side will work too. When your top arm is extended out, you will feel your lats down the side of your upper back on that side.

Single Leg Hip Extensions

1. Lie on your back and place one foot elevated on a chair or a lounge so that your upper and lower leg are forming a right angle. (The further you are away from that object the harder it will be.) The second leg hangs in the air either straight up or bent, whatever is comfortable for you.
2. Lift your hips in the air as high as your flexibility allows. Make sure you squeeze your butt when you get towards the top of the movement.
3. Lower your leg and make sure your butt stays off the ground each

time. Ensure that your other leg doesn't touch the ground. Repeat for the desired number of repetitions then swap legs.

- Where should you feel it?
Your hamstrings in the back of your legs and your butt in the leg that is working. The leg that's in the air is resting in this exercise. The higher you lift your hips the more you will likely feel it in your quads in the front of your thighs and your abs.

Ski Jumps
1. Stand with your feet shoulder width apart.
2. Jump both feet together sideways in a comfortable jump about 3-5cm or so making sure you are landing on the balls of your feet. You don't want to over exaggerate this movement.

3. Repeat that motion, jumping back across to the other side and landing on the balls of your feet again.
4. Jumping left then right (or vice versa) counts as two in your count.

- Where should you feel it?
This is a cardio exercise designed to get your heart rate up in limited space. Your calf muscles (backs of your lower legs) will feel it a little bit too.

Spiderman Twists
1. Start with your hands on the ground and hold yourself up on your toes (a starting regular push up position), making sure your back is as parallel to the ground as you can get it.
2. Twist one leg across your body towards your opposite shoulder as far as your flexibility allows.
3. Bring that leg back and repeat with the other leg twisting across to the opposite shoulder (or as far as you can) for the desired number of repetitions. Make sure you keep your speed slow and controlled.

- Where should you feel it?
Your abs and your obliques (sides of the midsection) are the primary muscles working here. You may also feel your shoulders and arms a little because they're supporting your body. The front of the thighs and inner thighs may also switch on a little bit too.

Split Squats
1. Place one leg behind your body, resting on your toes. Place your front leg flat on the ground in front of your body at a comfortable stance with your foot pointing straight ahead.
2. Bend both knees making sure that all the weight of the front leg is

driving down through your front heel. You don't want your knee going too far forward over your toes.

3. Your back knee will move down towards the ground when you bend your front leg and lower as far as you can before raising and repeating the movement for as many repetitions as necessary.

4. Hold on to something if you can't keep your balance. Try to look at something straight ahead or put your finger in your belly button to help you balance (this sounds silly but it works surprisingly well).

5. Switch legs for the next exercise to work the opposite muscles to those you've just worked.

- Where should you feel it?

When you drive down through your front heel you'll feel it work deeper in the front of your back thigh (quads) and in your front leg you'll feel your hamstrings (back of the leg) and your glutes.

Sprinters Shuffles

1. Start with your hands on the ground and hold yourself up on your toes (a starting regular push up position), making sure your back is as parallel to the ground as you can get it.

2. Drive one leg straight ahead towards your shoulders as far as your flexibility allows.

3. Bring that leg back and repeat with the other leg for the desired number of repetitions. Make sure you keep your speed slow and controlled.

4. The movement is similar to a Spiderman Twist, except this time you are not twisting across your body, just driving straight up and down.

- Where should you feel it?

Your abs are the primary muscles working here. You may also feel your shoulders and arms a little because they're supporting your body. The front of the thighs may also switch on a little bit too.

Squat and Drive

1. Stand with your legs just outside shoulder width apart.

2. Squat down, making sure as you are lowering your body, you're placing the weight of your body through your heels.

3. The best way to do this is to imagine you're sitting down on a chair that's further back than you expected. Or start the movement by pushing your butt backwards.

4. Squat down as far as you can comfortably go, making sure your knees don't come too far forward. Don't let them go past your knees.

5. As you're starting to stand up, drive one leg up and rise off the ground.

6. Squat down for your next repetition and lift your other leg as you stand up. Complete as many repetitions as necessary. The movement is like what you'd imagine a sumo wrestler would do when they do their little pre-wrestle dance.

- Where should you feel it?
The quads in the front of your thighs as well as your butt and in the back of thighs. When you drive up in the movement your butt and hamstrings will work a little bit more than in a normal Squat.

Step Body Blasts
1. Start standing up and bend down placing both your hands in front of you on a small elevation like a step.
2. Jump your legs back together behind you so your back is as close to parallel to the ground as you can get. Avoid your hips sagging down towards the floor.
3. Jump your legs apart at the same time.
4. Jump your legs back together, then jump them forward so they're just in front of your hands.
5. Stand up and repeat for as many repetitions as needed.
6. If this feels relatively easy, take out the step and do the Body Blasts with your hands on the ground. If it is too hard or you have had back issues previously, just walk your legs back and walk them apart instead of using the more explosive jumping movement.
7. You could also do this off something higher like a chair or lounge if you are a beginner.

- Where should you feel it?
This is a great cardio exercise so you should be puffed. The goal is to work up to doing these as quickly as you can while keeping your form. Draw your belly button in to avoid your lower back switching on and hurting.

Step Leg Shuffles
1. As per the regular Leg Shuffle, stand with your feet about shoulder width apart.
2. The difference with this variation is you're going to be doing the Leg Shuffles on a step that isn't too high - like the height of a gutter or a step in your home.
3. Keep your weight on the balls of your feet and shift your legs back and forwards like you're moving your feet in a scissor movement.
4. Remember that back and forwards counts as two repetitions in this instance. Complete as many repetitions as necessary.

- Where should you feel it?

Mainly a great cardio exercise designed to get your heart rate up. The step adds to the intensity of the movement and you'll feel it more in your calf muscles compared to the regular version.

NOTE: If your back doesn't like this version, just use the regular Leg Shuffle or an alternate cardio exercise demonstrated in these pages.

Stick Ups

1. Stand up straight with your arms extended above your head.
2. Lower your arms down so your fingers are almost at the level of your shoulders.
3. As you're lowering your arms, squeeze your shoulder blades together (I like to imagine there's something in between the shoulder blades that I'm trying to touch when I squeeze them together).
4. Extend your arms as far as possible back above your head to the starting position and repeat for desired number of repetitions.

- Where should you feel it?

Your lat muscles that run down the sides of your upper back and your trapezius in your upper back.

Stick Ups with Calf Raises

1. Follow the same steps for the regular Stick Ups.
2. The only difference here is as you extend your arms back above your head to complete the Stick Up movement, stand up on your toes to engage the calf muscles. Then lower your arms and your heels down to the ground at the same time. Complete as many repetitions as necessary.

- Where should you feel it?

Same spots as for a regular Stick Up in your lats and traps plus you'll feel your calf muscles with the raises.

Up and Overs

1. Sit on the ground with an object like an upended foam roller or a large water bottle placed just in front of your legs.
2. Starting with your legs on one side, lift your legs in the air and lift them up and over the object and come back. Repeat for the desired number of repetitions.
3. For beginners start with your knees bent. To make it harder straighten your legs until you hit the point where it's the right intensity for you.
4. Your hands can support you on the ground, or if you need extra lower back support, you can lie back on your forearms or even flat on your back.

5. The lower your legs come towards the ground, without actually touching it, the harder it is. Complete as many repetitions as necessary.
6. If you feel it in your lower back, just bend your knees a little bit more and don't come down as low.

- Where should you feel it?
All through your abs and your oblique muscles in the sides of your midsection.

Virtual Skipping
1. You can use a rope if you have one, or if you struggle with getting into a constant momentum because you keep breaking your jump when your feet catch the rope, or if you don't have a rope, go the virtual option.
2. Skipping without a rope can actually be harder because you can't break your rhythm and get to focus on the movement rather than constantly re-setting and starting again.
3. Place your arms out by your sides as if you were holding an actual skipping rope and move your wrists and forearms as you jump.
4. Make sure you land lightly on the balls of your feet. Complete as many repetitions as necessary.

- Where should you feel it?
A cardio exercise designed to get your heart rate up. You may feel it in your calves too.

V Sit Hold
1. Sit on the ground and lift your legs up in the air.
2. Hold for the allocated number of seconds in the workout. Rest if your lower back starts to hurt then resume if there's still time left.
3. The straighter your legs are, the harder it is. If you're a beginner, or feel it in your lower back, experiment with having your knees anywhere from totally bent to just slightly bent to make it harder.
4. If you need support for your lower back, you can rest on your forearms or with your hands on the ground. It's harder if you're not holding on and have your arms by your side.
5. If that's easy, you can extend your arms out so they are parallel to the ground or extend them above your head for even more of a challenge.

- Where should you feel it?
Your abs. If you feel it in your lower back, you may need to modify your position and not have your legs as low to the ground. Draw in your belly button to stop this from happening.

Waiters Bows
1. Make sure your knees are slightly bent, not locked out, to take the strain away from your lower back.
2. Bend your back at the waist so you're pushing your butt behind you as you bend forward.
3. Keep looking straight ahead to keep your back straight. The depth you can bend forward will depend on your flexibility. Come down far enough to feel the back of your legs.
4. NOTE: Some people find their upper back rounds when they do this. If this is you (try doing it in front a mirror to see), really focus on pushing your butt back and keeping your shoulders back.

- Where should you feel it?
The backs of your legs (hamstrings) are the main area here and you will likely feel it in your butt too.

Wall Sit
1. Stand in front of a wall with enough room to rest your back against it when you're holding a squat position.
2. Squat down to a position that's effective for you by sliding your back down the wall. Ideally, you want your thighs as close to parallel to the ground as you can. But if you're a beginner, you won't need to come down as far.
3. Hold for the allocated number of seconds in the workout.
4. Make sure your knees follow the angle of your feet without extending over your toes.
5. This exercise should be okay even if you have bad knees because you only have to set your knees in position once and you may even want to use it as a substitution for other squat exercises in this book.

- Where should you feel it?
Mainly in the front of your thighs (quads) but the back of your legs (hamstrings) and butt (glutes) will also see some action.

Waves
1. Sit on the ground with your knees bent.
2. Place your hands by your sides and lift your hips up. Your hand position is up to you, but as per the Backstrokers, I like to have my hands facing forwards or I sometimes do them on my knuckles.
3. Hold your hips off the ground so your thighs are as close to parallel to the ground as possible.
4. Lift one arm up in the air above your head and alternate with the other arm for the desired number of repetitions.

- Where should you feel it?

Definitely backs of your arms (triceps) and shoulders. The higher in the air your hips are, the more you'll feel it in your abs and the quads in the front of your thighs.

Resources

You don't need any equipment to do the exercises in this workout program. But, if you find any of them easy, you may want to use a piece of equipment to add to the intensity of the exercise. It makes your body work harder.

If you use a foam roller, during abs exercises for example, by placing your forearms on one in the hover position, your body works harder to maintain stability. You can even use your roller for push-ups by placing your feet on one, or, if you have two, a hand on each one.

You can find the direct links for most of the products listed below on the book's resources page on the website

dpmworkout.com

They are not affiliate links and I don't make any commission out of recommending these to you. These are products that I recommend and personally use. (Prices are correct at time of publication).

Timer App:
What for? The workouts all use a timer so you're going to need a timer app on your phone. You can download one for free in your app store or follow along with the full-length videos that you can purchase as part of the DPM All-In package on the book's download page.

Price? I use Interval Timer Pro and it costs $4.49 in the app store. You can use the app to customise all your different timer options.

Alternatively, you could go with a free app but be prepared for ads and limited availability to pre-program new options.

Exercise Mat
What for? Perfect if you don't have any carpet. It's a bit more forgiving on the knees too. You could also use a towel if you don't have one.

Price? $5 to $8 from Kmart, depending on the thickness you'd prefer.

Skipping Rope
What for? Cardio.

Price: Buy the 2.7m speed rope at Kmart for $2. It's better than the more expensive ones I've tried.
Remember, stick to virtual skipping if you're stopping and re-starting

while using a rope. It'll be more effective because you'll keep your heart rate up.

Mini Exercise Bands
What for? To increase the intensity of exercises like Leg Shuffles, Side Lunges and Monster Walks. They can be placed just above your ankles or, to increase the intensity of Squats, they can be placed just above your knees.

Price: Ranging in price from $4.95 to $9.50 depending on the strength. The harder the resistance, the more expensive they are.

Foam Rollers
What for? I use one to add intensity to different exercises. Foam rollers can also be used to help release tension in your back and other parts of your body. I love laying long ways (from the top of your head down to your tailbone) to release all the tension in your vertebrae along your spine. Also great for hitting any other part of your body i.e. ITB's or thighs and lower back.

Price: Up to $39.90 depending on length.

Massage Balls
What for? Perfect for loosening up tight muscles. They act as a trigger point massage on your targeted area. To use them on your upper back for example, lie on your back and place the ball under your problem area. Use it just like you would a foam roller.

Price: $17.60. Kmart have them cheaper, but I can't verify their quality.

Boxing Gloves
What for? To give you extra weight resistance for your shadow boxing component of the workouts.

Price: $110 for my personal choice – Punch Equipment Trophy Getters. You can choose between 8oz to 18oz-weighted gloves, going up in 2oz or 4oz increments. The heavier the gloves, the more of a workout you'll get.

Yes, these gloves are expensive and you don't have to spend that much, or even buy any at all. You could just use your hands for the shadow boxing component. Obviously you can get weighted gloves for less but these are the best in the business and full leather, meaning they'll last longer and are the ones I use at DPM.

Kettlebells

What for? To increase the intensity of exercises by adding extra resistance. Examples include Squats, or to turn Waiters Bows into Deadlifts. You could also use for V Sit Holds to make them harder. These aren't necessary, but if you find certain exercises easy, then you could go down this avenue.

Price: Varies depending on weight, with the price increasing, as the weight gets heavier. As for where to buy them, you can find them anywhere from Kmart to Rebel or online these days. Find one that works for you, and your budget, as I don't have a preferred supplier.

The Best Advice I Can Offer You

I'll give it to you straight up. Short 'N Sweet.

Part 1:

The best time to start taking care of yourself by starting to eat better and exercise more was years ago. The next best time, if you obviously missed that boat, is NOW. Don't put it off any longer.

No matter how 'bad' your past may have been. You can build new habits. You have the power to act.

Part 2:

Do it.

Do what you said you would do.

If you said you'd start, then start. Don't just talk about it. Even if starting means making small changes. Maybe it's cutting out the wine or two with dinner every night to every other night, or just weekends.

Or maybe it's deciding to eat a little better each day. Or adding in a daily walk, or starting a workout program like this one. It's a start. Whatever you decide to focus on is progress.

Do what you said you would do.

Make sense? Sure, it's simple advice. But it's 100% spot on.

If you need help to get started, that's what the DPM All-In package, or training with me in person, is all about.

What's Next? How About The Full DPM All-In Package

If you want to take your training experience to another level to ensure that you get started and begin to lose your stubborn kilos, sign-up for the DPM All-In package.

What you'll get access to:

* Every single full length workout video included in Short 'N Sweet (six in total) plus six months' access to the accompanying DPM Online Training app via Trainerize ($294 separately.)

The customised app uploads each month's workouts for you. All you have to do is click on the workout and press play.

* PLUS you'll get the video URL link to watch on my hosted Vimeo page and I'll give you a link to download each video in my special Dropbox folder in .mp4 format. ($99 separately.)

* The DPM 6 Week Re-Set System comprising of 42 daily emails with a simple mission each day as well as the full food plan and my Quick, Healthy Meals recipe book ($97 separately.)

The Re-Set program's explained in more detail on the next page.

That's $490 in total value but I'll give you a real incentive to grab it and help you actually follow through and complete this book and enjoy the results.

You can have all of that for a once-off investment of only $247!

And, as for everything in this book, you can access that at dpmworkout.com

The DPM 6 Week Re-Set Online System

Would you like to train with DPM but are cursing yourself because you don't live locally? Well, I've got your back.

The DPM 6 Week Re-Set Online System (included in the DPM All-In Package) is for you.

You'll get a daily email containing one simple step to follow for that particular day. This approach breaks down a six-week process into a simple day-by-day action list.

It takes away the confusion that can often arise when you start a new program.

This online program is different. Follow the steps every day and you simply can't go wrong.

You'll also get access to the full game plan, which I recommend you follow as well to the best of your capabilities.

And that full game plan? How about the results-producing DPM 3 Day Detox Diet and the DPM Quick, Healthy Meals recipe book (giving you great tasting meals that the kids will even enjoy in 20 minutes or less).

You'll also get a new bonus workout to follow. All of these bonuses are available via instant PDF and excel download once your investment is confirmed.

That 'Detox Diet' by the way, doesn't require you to drink some silly syrup or take something dangerous. It's just a three-day break from processed carbs. This simple process works a treat.

You may be wondering how much all of this will set you back? I've sold this separately for $97, but it's all included in your DPM All-In Package.

Got a question? Send me an email and I'll do my best to get back to you within 24-hours - daniel@dpmtransformation.com

Or Maybe You'd Prefer To Train With Me In Person?

If you'd like to train with me, there are a couple of options available. DPM early morning small group sessions are currently held at Lilyfield in Sydney's Inner West and Observatory Hill in the CBD.

You can even have two weeks on the house to ensure that we're both a good fit for each other and to prove that DPM is the right solution for you.

Or you can choose DPM one-on-one personal training. It's held in the same spots and at other select locations in Sydney (in your home or outdoors at a local park).

If none of those are appropriate, the final option is DPM Online Coaching. I'll design a customised program for you that you can easily access via the Trainerize app, complete with demonstration videos.

You'll also have me check-in with you via email weekly or daily via SMS (depending on your package) to make sure you're on track.

All you have to do is fill in the form below and I'll be in touch within 24-hours.

https://dpmperformance.wufoo.com/forms/interested-in-finding-out-more-about-dpm-training/

Alternatively, if all that seems like too much hard work typing all that into your browser, then email me - daniel@dpmtransformation.com and let me know what you're looking for.

My Shout For Dinner?

There's one more thing I'll mention. How does a free dinner for you and your partner sound? All you have to do is refer a friend of yours to join us at DPM.

Once they've been training with DPM at either our small group or one-on-one personal training options for only six months, I'll shout you both a $200 dinner gift card to any restaurant of your choice.

There's no fine print or exclusions. You'll get one, and your friend who joins will get one too as a thank you for trusting me as your training solution. And if it's your partner who joins, then you double up and get two different vouchers, or one big $400 one!

This promotion has proven to be very popular amongst DPMers and the best part is there's no limit to how many vouchers you can receive.

If you have encouraged three friends to join, and they all do once they've finished their two weeks free test-drive, you'll get three free dinner vouchers for $200 each once their six month anniversary comes along.

I'll contact you and ask you where you want to eat. And I'll do the same for your friends too so they can make the most of theirs. That's all there is to it.

And another incentive that you don't have to wait six months to enjoy, for every friend of yours who does join DPM on your recommendation, you'll receive your next month on the house as a thank you.

For those who are currently not training with DPM, but still encourage someone to join, I'll shout you a $100 VISA gift card instead.

Just make sure that your friend drops your name when they contact me and mention this promotion!

About Me

I am a Body Transformation Specialist based in Sydney, with a Bachelor of Health Science (PD/H/PE major) as well as being a Certificate 3 and 4 qualified personal trainer.

I've been in the fitness industry since 2000 and have been helping busy women (and a few blokes too) through my DPM Performance personal training business since 2005.

DPM specialises in short, interval driven, weight loss programs that usually helps busy mums finally lose their 'mummy tummy' and get back in the skinny jeans that have been hiding at the back of their wardrobe. The guys usually just want to keep in shape so they can still enjoy a few beers.

Outside of work, I've been married to Bronwyn since 2009 and my greatest accomplishment is being a proud Dad to Emily and Jade, the best job in the world!

Over the last decade I've created a bunch of different online training systems with the current focus being the DPM 6 Week Re-Set Blueprint and Busy Mums 4 Week Transformation System. These follow-along-at-home training programs give busy people the results they deserve in only three short 20-minute workouts each week.

You'll also discover that you don't have to live on rabbit food with the easy to follow food plans that still let you enjoy your favourite drink and treat foods, just like I do.

Once you start training the DPM way, you'll have more energy, be more alert, more productive at work, and be more present with your kids. Your family and friends will love the new you.

Don't be surprised when they start accusing you of 'having work done'. More importantly, you'll love the new you that stares back at you in the mirror each day.

It just leaves the final question - Why not you?

Daniel Munday
DPM Performance
w: dpmtransformation.com
w: dpmworkout.com
e: daniel@dpmtransformation.com